Beginner Pole Dancing

For Fitness and Fun

By

Danni Peck

Beginner Pole Dancing: For Fitness and Fun

Copyright © 2017

All rights reserved. This book or any portion thereof may not be reproduced or used in any manner whatsoever without the express written permission of the publisher except for the use of brief quotations in a book review.

ISBN-10: 1521190755

ISBN-13: 978-1521190753

Warning and Disclaimer

Every effort has been made to make this book as accurate as possible. However, no warranty or fitness is implied. The information provided is on an "as-is" basis. The author and the publisher shall have no liability or responsibility to any person or entity with respect to any loss or damages that arise from the information in this book.

Publisher contact

Skinny Bottle Publishing

books@skinnybottle.com

Introduction to Pole Dancing	1
What You Need to Begin Pole Dancing	2
A Pole	2
Clothes Matter	3
Oils and Pole Grip	4
Stretching	4
You'll Feel Sore	5
The Wrap Around	6
A Basic Climb	8
The Fireman Spin	12
How to Do Beginner Slides	15
Back Slide	16
Leg Squat Slide	18
Bunny Slide	20
Lunging Slide	22
Shoulder Slide	24
Thread the Needle	26
Transitional Moves and How to Do Them	28
What are Transitional Moves	28
Body Wave	29
Backwards Wiggle	29
Pole Wiggles	30
Hip Circles	31
Pole Frisking	32
Knee Bridge	34
Shoulder Bridge	36

Clock Legs	38
Log Roll	40
More Beginner Moves to Perfect and Learn	**42**
Hook Spin	42
Martini	44
Chair Spin	46
Pike Spin	48
Back Hook Spin	50
Stag Spin	52
Crucifix Climb	54
Go Shine!	**56**

Introduction to Pole Dancing

Pole dancing is an exercise that's been sweeping the nation as of late! Every day, tons of men and women engage in this amazing and fun activity. You might want to try pole dancing as well but upon seeing some of the moves, you might not think you're able to do it.

The truth is, anyone can learn how to pole dance and anyone can do this in a self-taught manner. This book will guide you through all of the beginning techniques to learn pole dancing. For many, learning pole dancing can be quite scary, and for some, that fear might hold them back. But this book will walk you through the exact basics you need to know about pole dancing, in order to really master it. You don't need to have prior dancing experience, or even strength; because you'll condition your body to before you begin.

Now, you could go to a studio, but this book will teach you everything you need to master a few of the beginner moves to become the best beginner pole dancer you can be.

What You Need to Begin Pole Dancing

There are a few things you should have before beginning your pole dancing journey. This chapter will discuss them and why they are necessary.

A Pole

Well, you need a pole to pole dance, right? If you're pole dancing at a studio, choose one pole that you'll be using for the duration of your training and conditioning. If you're doing this at home, getting a free-standing pole is the best option.

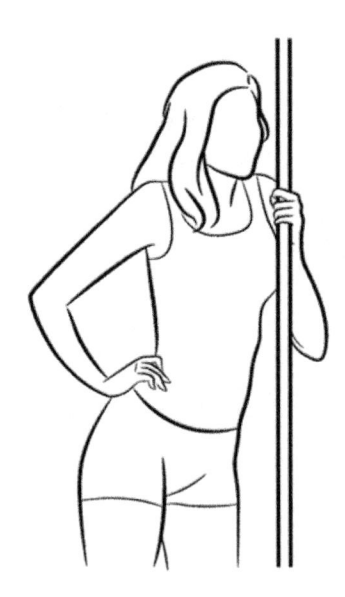

Now, there are two types of poles — static and spinning. You can also get one that does both. Ultimately, if you want to learn more advanced techniques, you'll want to get a pole that spins. But for a beginner, using one that has both functions is ideal. For learning the beginner moves, you can use a static one;

just realize that it'll require more direct upper body strength since you can't use the momentum of the pole with a static pole.

Now, a VERY important part, and I won't stress this enough, is do NOT cheap out when buying a pole. If you feel like you might not commit to this right away, see if there's a place where you can try out a pole — such as a pole studio that has a free dance — or even a friend. Typically, a good pole runs about $300. You shouldn't go to an adult entertainment store and get one of those. You know those pole fail videos on the Internet? Those are caused by a cheap pole. I highly recommend an X-pole, because not only does that brand give you detailed instructions, there are also great how-to videos on this subject as well.

Once you get the pole, if you're buying one to use at home, set it up per the instructions. Make sure it is secured to the top of the crossbeams of your house. If not, the pole will move and that creates a safety hazard that could injure you.

You should make sure that you're doing this on a soft floor. A carpet typically absorbs most of the blows. However, if you are attempting pole dancing on a hardwood surface try to have some cushioning against the bottom, especially if you're learning the more difficult inverted moves and spins. Falling on your head is never fun, that's for sure.

Once you have that setup, it's time for the next part of pole dancing, your clothing.

Clothes Matter

Now, lots of people give pole dancing a bad name because it's always associated with strippers. Yes, strippers did popularize this method of dancing but anyone can do it these days. You might see a lot of girls who pole dance wearing practically nothing. This isn't just to show off their curves, (of course, some might be doing it for that reason), but there is a practical reason behind this.

You need to wear clothing that doesn't cover much because your body's friction is how you'll grip the pole. If you wear clothes, they will create a slippery surface and that's how people fall. Do not wear pants unless they're the pole gripping pants some retailers sell, and if you want leggings like that, they are nice to wear. Ideally, you should wear a sports bra and some shorts that aren't too long. For performance reasons, some pole dancers wear fancier bras and underwear. You can also wear cotton panties as well if you're at home.

When it comes to heels, you can wear them. It often is a means to feeling sexier, and some pole dancers like the extra height that heels give them. Wearing heels almost forces you to point your toes out. But it's not necessary. You can pole dance barefoot to help with grip at first, especially when learning new moves.

Do not try to overdress for learning pole dancing; it is a great way to help build body confidence. If you've been feeling like you don't look good enough for it, don't worry about it. Remember, you're doing this for you.

Oils and Pole Grip

Now, before you begin this, you should not wear body lotions. Simply put, the oils from the lotion will transfer to the pole and will make it slick, causing you to slip and fall down. If you tend to wear lotion, skip applying in on the days you're going to pole dance and you won't risk the potential of falling.

However, there is something called pole grip. You might not need this right away because it can be a bit pricey, but you can rub it into your skin and it creates a gripping surface. This is great for when you begin practicing more complex moves and you tend to sweat a lot. It'll help keep your grip. You can buy this on Amazon if you so desire. A small jar is about 12 bucks, but it lasts a long time.

Stretching

Now, remember that pole dancing is like any other forms of exercise, in that you need to stretch out your body. This is also important for later when you try to do some of the more complex moves. A tight leg might be the difference between you landing that move or not. A light stretch and a bit of a warm-up will help. You can touch your toes, stretch out your arms by pulling them over your elbow and holding, and even doing neck and shoulder rolls to get the kinks out. You can also pull your leg back to your butt to give you a nice stretch in your hamstring. Obviously, the stretching isn't limited to that but ideally you should get at least a little stretch in before you begin pole dancing.

A big part of stretching is of your hands. Many dancers forget this part but it's integral to stretch out your wrists and hands. You can do this by gripping your fingers with the palms facing outward and holding it. You should feel a stretch in the wrist area. This will make gripping the pole that much easier.

When some pole dancers are warming up, they'll do some of the beginner moves before they tackle some of the more advanced ones. For the purpose of this beginner book, you'll just do these stretches before learning the basics.

You'll Feel Sore

Just as a heads up — and some people already know this — but once you begin pole dancing, you're going to feel sore. Often, most people don't feel this sore even when they're in shape. Pole dancing works out parts of your body you're not used to and some of the bruises that you get can get quite nasty. Make sure that you go into this knowing that you'll probably regret everything the next day. Just remember: The gains and skill are worth all the pain. And while it might hurt quite a bit initially, once you get used to this and start to condition those areas of your body, it gets much easier.

Having these stretches and moves in your repertoire before you begin will allow a safe and fun pole dancing experience.

The Wrap Around

This is the first move that you'll learn when beginning pole dancing. This chapter will go over just how you do this in a concise, and exact manner.

To begin, stand behind your pole, with the inside of your dominant foot at the closer end of the pole. If you're a righty, that means right and vice versa. You should have your dominant hand grab the pole right where your head is. Allow your arm to straighten up a little bit so that you can feel the weight of your body almost hanging away from the pole.

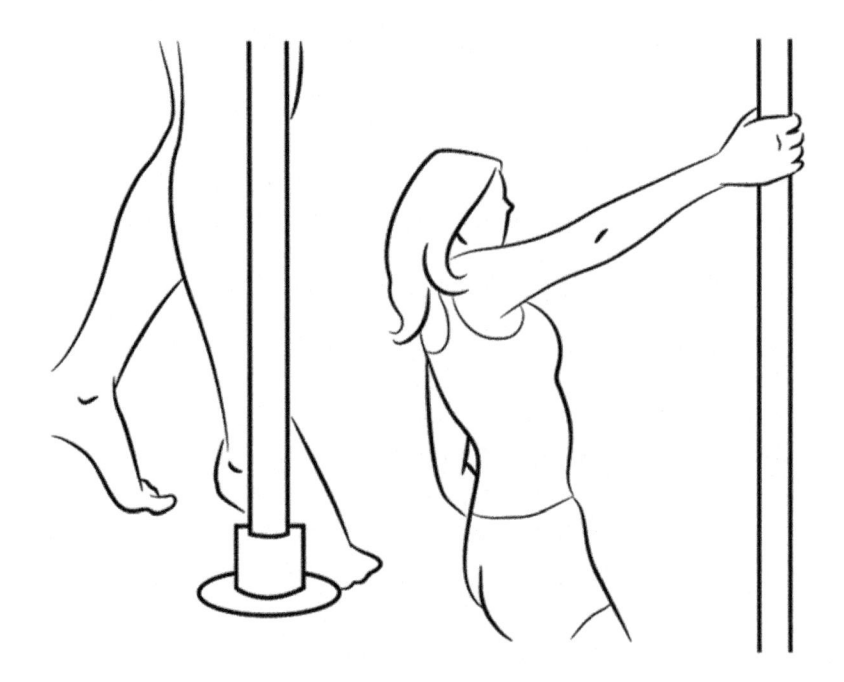

Now, you should take your outside leg (the one that isn't nearest the pole), keep it straight, then swing it towards the outside and have it go all the way around the pole. You will feel your inside foot start to pivot at this time as well. While doing this, you should have the knee bent slightly and not locked straight, since it'll make it look much more graceful. You should strive to keep your toes pointed as well.

Next, you begin to hook the pole area with your dominant foot. To do this, you should take your outside foot and put it behind the other foot. Take your weight and put it on the back foot allowing you to hook your dominant leg around the front area of your pole, having the grip right behind the knee.

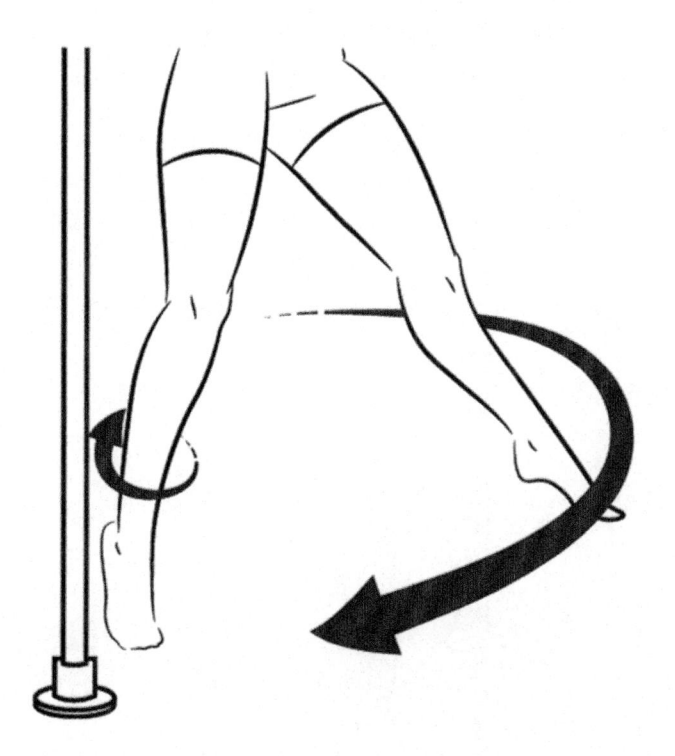

, to finish off this move and to make it look sexy, arch your upper body and place your hand on the pole at about chest level in to create a better arch. Now, to help improve your flexibility, you should arch your upper body as far back as you feel comfortable and have most of the weight and grip on the leg and hand around the pole. Hold this and you'll even feel a small stretch. This is a fun and sexy beginner move for those looking to try something different.

You can then put your leg down and get back to your straight posture. You should then grip the pole to begin the next move. This is a great transitional move into harder moves, but it's also great for beginners to learn.

A Basic Climb

Pole dancing is often known for two types of moves: Spins and climbs. Fortunately, beginners can do these as well. This chapter will go over how you can do the basic climb and allow you to finally get off the ground and onto the pole.

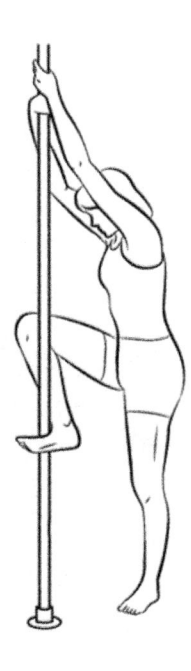

Now, the first thing to learn is that this can be a bit scary. Often, when a person is learning pole dancing, it's a bit anxiety-inducing to be off the ground. Even a simple climb such as this one can be scary. (I used to be afraid of leaving the ground.) But remember, practice makes perfect! This is one of the moves that might take a moment to get used to, but as you continue to practice, your anxiety will lessen, and you'll be able to master it.

To begin, you should have your body directly at the pole. You should be about a foot or so away from it when looking at it. You should then grip the pole with your dominant hand first.

From there, you should take the dominant leg and bring it up to the pole while you grip the pole. You should have the pole around your foot, flexing your foot slightly. Your knee should be on the other side of where your foot is. You should feel it almost anchor itself there, which is what you need to pull yourself up. If you don't, you'll fall, so make sure that this is sturdy before you do the next part.

Once you've got the anchor there, you should then pull yourself up using your hands, taking the leg that you still have on the ground and putting it behind your other leg. Put the knee of the leg you just raised on the other side of the pole, allowing you to have a grip there with your knees. By doing this, you've created a platform with your legs to begin climbing the pole, which is what we'll go over in a later chapter. Now, it might seem awkward to you for a second, because you're holding your body up and this is where the strength training comes in. By doing this more and more, you'll be able to pull your body up with ease, until it's almost second nature.

You can then take your hands and move them a foot up on the pole so that they can be straightened. You'll then use your abs to help pull your knees up a foot or so, keeping the knees bent to help grip. You shouldn't move your feet, but instead, use your abs and the grip of your legs to propel yourself.

Once you've done the climb, you can then lean your body back a bit, holding the pole with your leg muscles and straightening them as you continue to climb up the pole. Essentially, you'll continue to do this to climb higher, until you reach your comfort level. You'll certainly feel the workout and you can even hold it there for a minute or so to feel it as well. If you're afraid of heights, inching up on the pole a little bit at a time does wonders and it'll make it much easier and less scary for you!

Now, to come off the pole, you can slide down from it by loosening yourself slightly, or you can grip the pole with your hands, release your legs for a second, put them in front of your body and move your hips and legs down to the ground. Obviously, you should also move your hands as well to help you get down. This does take a bit of getting used to, but once you master it, it'll make you look even better.

This climb is a great way to begin learning some of the more complicated actions. For many, it can take some time to feel comfortable and confident with this move and it can be scary. But upon learning it, you'll soon be a master in no time!

The Fireman Spin

This is the most basic spin to learn, but it's very sexy. Mastering it can certainly help you look even better and allow you to try more complex spins and moves.

To begin with this, you need to take your hands and hold the pole with them. You should stand next to the pole so it's closer to the weaker side of your body. Take your hands and grip the pole like a baseball bat but placed about a foot or so apart. The hand that is next to the pole should be on top and have the outside on the bottom. Keep the lower hand near where your eye level area is, but your other hand should be above your head.

You should then take a step with the foot near the pole and take the leg that is outside around. This will get momentum, and you'll feel your body start to speed up, enough to circle around the pole area. With this move, it's best to start with the pole in static mode if you can, so that you're not moving too fast and end up getting dizzy.

Next, with the momentum going, you should pull up against the pole so that your arms are supporting the entire weight of your body for a second. From there, push off and jump on the foot inside and then grab the pole with both of your knees. You should make sure that you're gripping the pole in a secure manner.

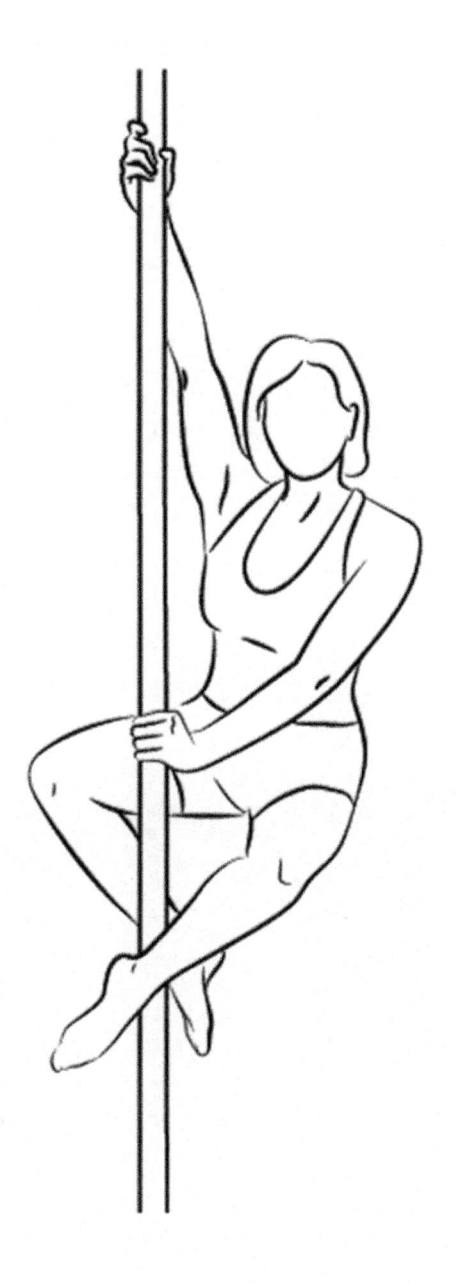

You'll then start spinning, and you can hold the pole in the similar climb position that was discussed earlier. You can also move your left leg a bit forward as well. Now, as a rule of thumb, the higher your arms are at the initial position, the longer you'll spin, so if you want a nice long spin, do try to keep them in the position mentioned without sacrificing your grip.

Now, once you've finished, you can then put your legs down, move your hips back and then put yourself in a standing position. From there, you can begin to do other transitional moves or other spins and climbs, which we'll get into a bit later.

The fireman spin is a fun one to help those who fear to getting off the ground. If you are also afraid of going fast, try this a couple of times in order to perfect it. If you want to go a bit faster; before you swing your outerleg around and move your inner leg to the pole, do a couple of steps around the pole first. This is a great way to get the momentum going and it can make the move look much sexier.

How to Do Beginner Slides

One sexy part of pole dancing is the slides that you can try. There are so many to choose from and lots of great beginner techniques that allow you to segue to transitional moves and even floor work. If you're looking to add to your combos (allowing you to have an even more fluid motion), then try out these beginner slides. They're super simple and they can make any pole dancing combo look even better.

Now you might wonder if there is a difference between a slide and transition, and in a sense, a slide is a form of transition but don't have as much hip rotation and gyration. Sliding against the pole can sometimes be hard to maintain, especially for a beginner. Often, controlling the movement of your legs up and down in this manner is the real trick. You'll learn a few slides in this chapter; enough to get you started and allow you to use them in your combinations as well.

Back Slide

A backslide is the first slide you should learn, and this might take a moment to get used to. Initially, you might feel as if you're falling, but don't freak out; instead try holding the pole, maintaining an exact grip as you do this. To start, you should have your back against the pole with both arms straight and holding the pole behind your body. You should begin with your body held straight. You can put one hand on top of the other or just place both at the same level. Take one leg and put it forward, keeping your toes completely pointed. You should then slide down while you start to bend your supporting leg. Ideally, choose the dominant leg to slide down while the weaker leg is there to hold. You might slip and fall at first, but if you work to maintain a slow, controlled motion, you should be fine.

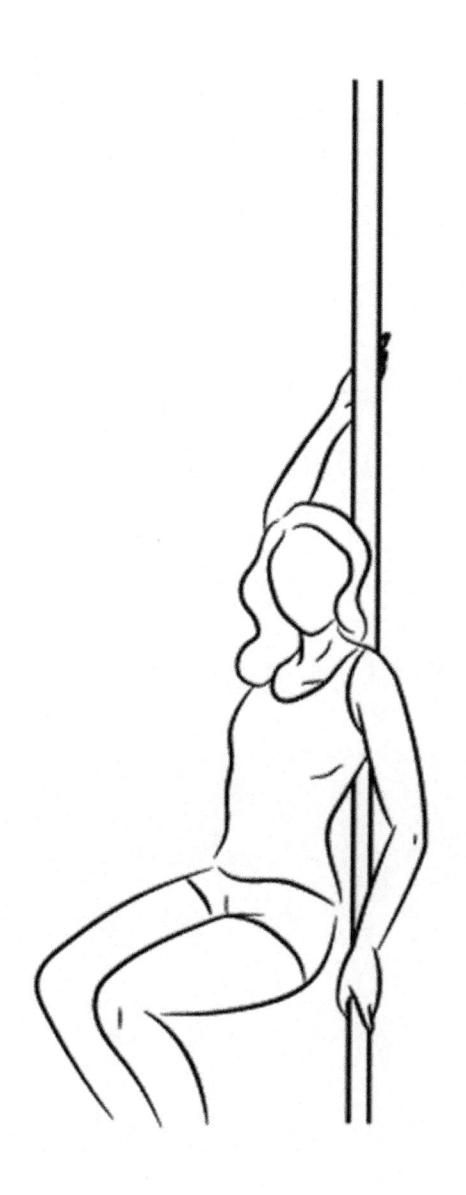

Leg Squat Slide

Now, if you like to do squats and want to incorporate them into your pole routine, well guess what? You can do this! This is a good move to help you feel the burn in your thighs and butt, while also allowing you to learn a sleek, sexy pole dancing move as well.

To begin, you should be in the same position as before, standing up straight with your back against the pole. However, move your legs out, spreading them apart, almost as far as you can. You should then start lowering your body, bending your knees as you begin to get into a squat position as you start to slide down. Once you've reached the level of comfort that you feel best with, you can then put your hands on your knees. If you want this to look sexy, you can hold onto the pole behind you while one hand is at your side. To get back up, simply move from the squat position up to the normal position you were in before, maybe gyrating your hips for an added sexy touch.

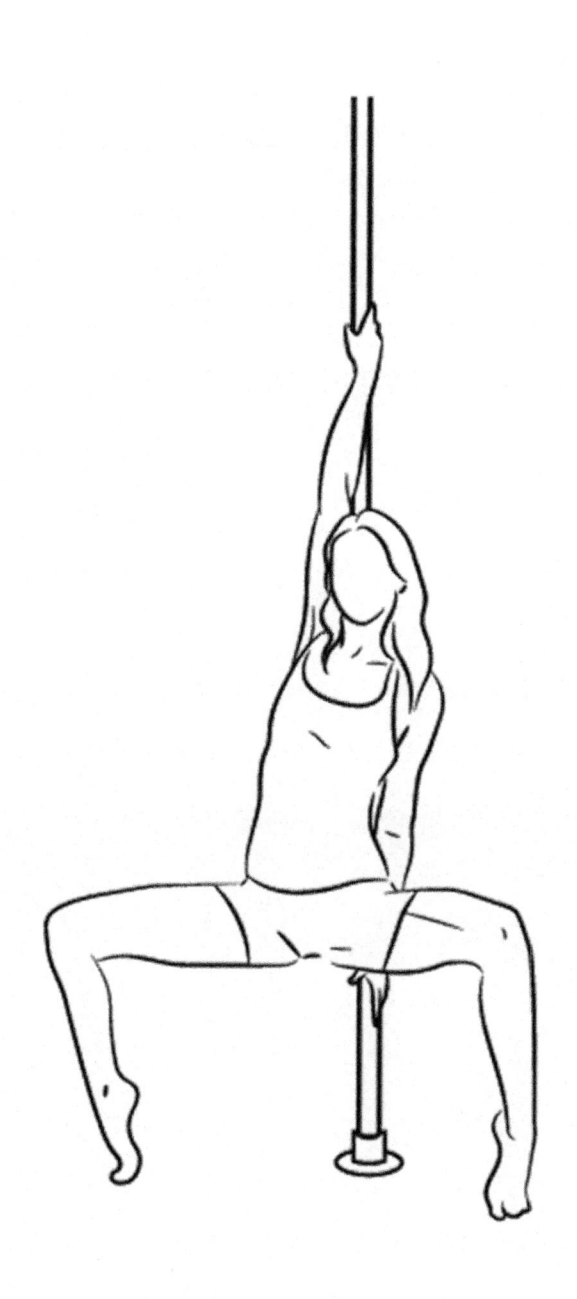

Bunny Slide

This is another simple pole slide but this time, you won't be touching the pole. This one is a more controlled and slower motion — the goal is to make this look fluid. Start by standing once again with your back against the pole and your arms on your thighs. Then, start to lower your thighs and slide down, getting into almost a crouched position. You'll certainly feel a thigh burn as you do this so make sure to take this slowly. You can grip the pole if you begin to feel your balance start falter because of this motion.

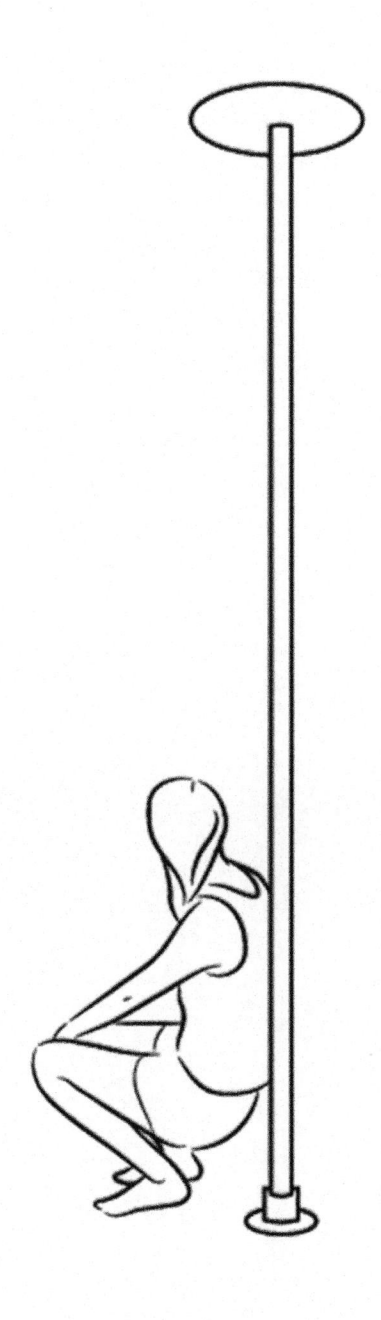

Lunging Slide

If you like lunges, then this is the slide for you! if you've ever done a curtsy lunge at the gym, this slide is very similar. You start by having your body straight with your back to the pole and one arm holding the pole. Make sure the arm is behind you, gripping it from behind almost above your head. You can take the other arm and either have it at your side or for more support, grab it right at your mid-back level. From there, take the opposite leg of your dominant hand and start to push it out towards the side of the pole. You should keep your toe that is being extended pointed as you slide down to a comfortable lunge level. You should keep your knee bent on the supporting leg. You can keep the supporting leg pointed as well, once you get familiar with the motion. To come back up from this, you simply bring that leg in and slide up.

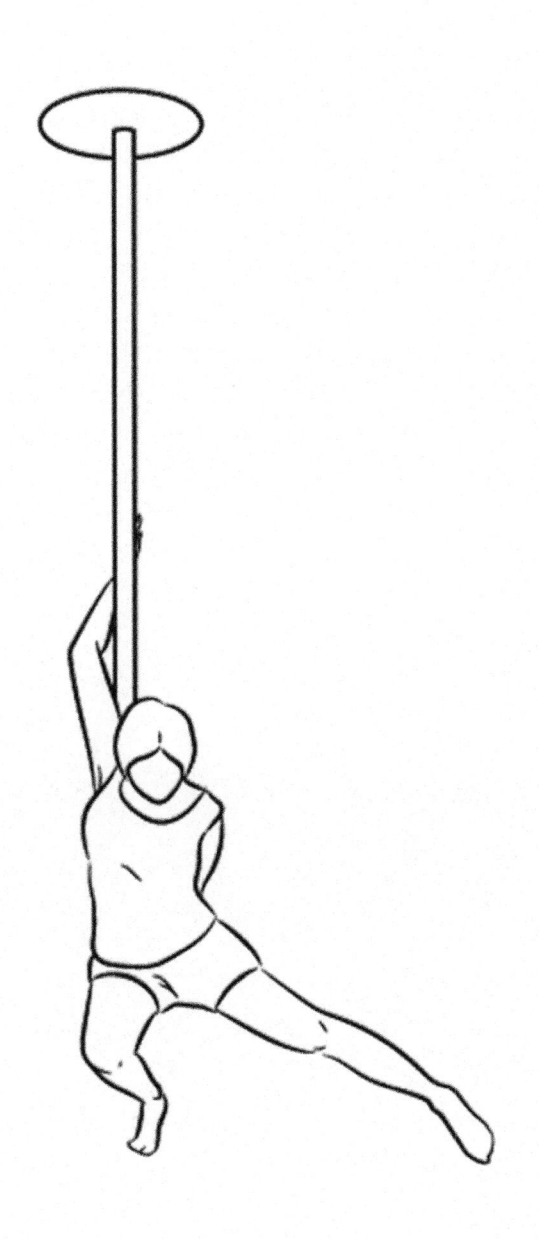

Shoulder Slide

This is a variation of the leg slide, but instead of just using your arms to brace you, most of the weight is on your shoulder. To begin, hold your body straight up with your back against the pole and both arms gripping the pole above your head behind you. Start to slide your feet as far forward as you possibly can, with one leg bent and the other leg straightened. You should have your shoulders resting against the pole. From that position, start to slide down on your shoulders in a controlled manner. Make sure to have one of your legs straight and one of them bent. Ideally, the dominant leg is the one that should be used to help support you initially, but you can practice with each leg as you go along. Make sure to keep your hips up and your back neutral as you do this, for it'll help to not only give you a good stretch, it'll also make the move much sexier.

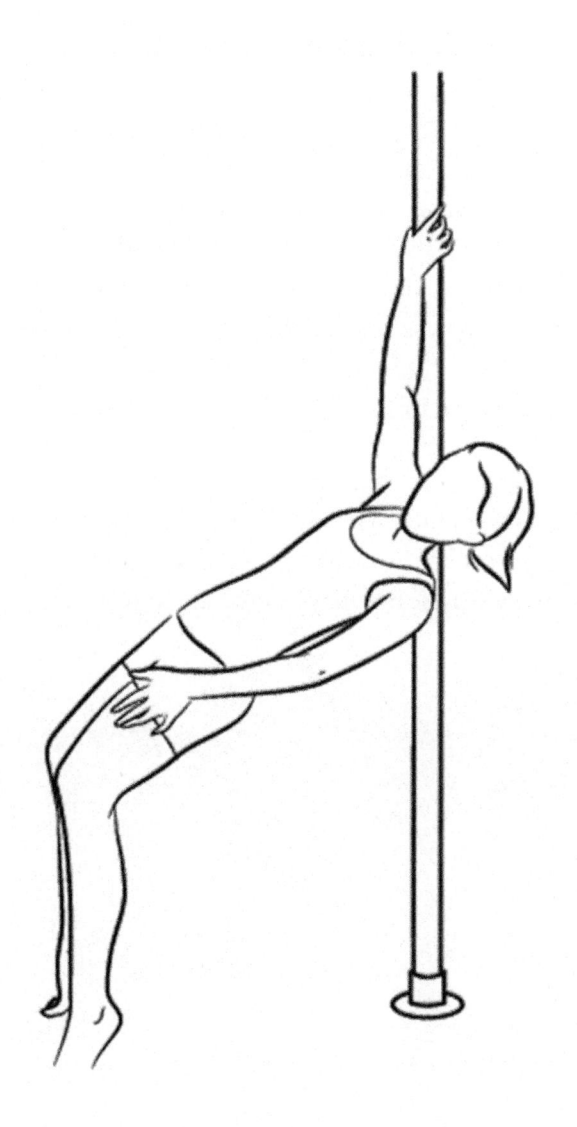

Thread the Needle

This is a variant of the lunge slide as previously mentioned. To do this, you should be in the standing position, once again with your back against the pole. You should have your arm hold the pole behind you. However, instead of just sliding your opposite leg out, you take the same leg as your hand and start to push it behind your other leg, sliding it out slightly. Now, you should keep your toes pointed, and the leg that isn't extended should be bent and supporting you. You can then slowly slide down the pole. This is probably the hardest slide mentioned in this chapter, so try to master the other ones, especially the lunge slide, before attempting this one. However, once you do this move, you'll realize just how pretty it looks.

These slides are a great way to help you build strength and give you a chance to learn controlled movements, while also keeping your toes pointed. Both of these skills are important to learn before you move onto harder moves, so take your time and practice these before you push forward.

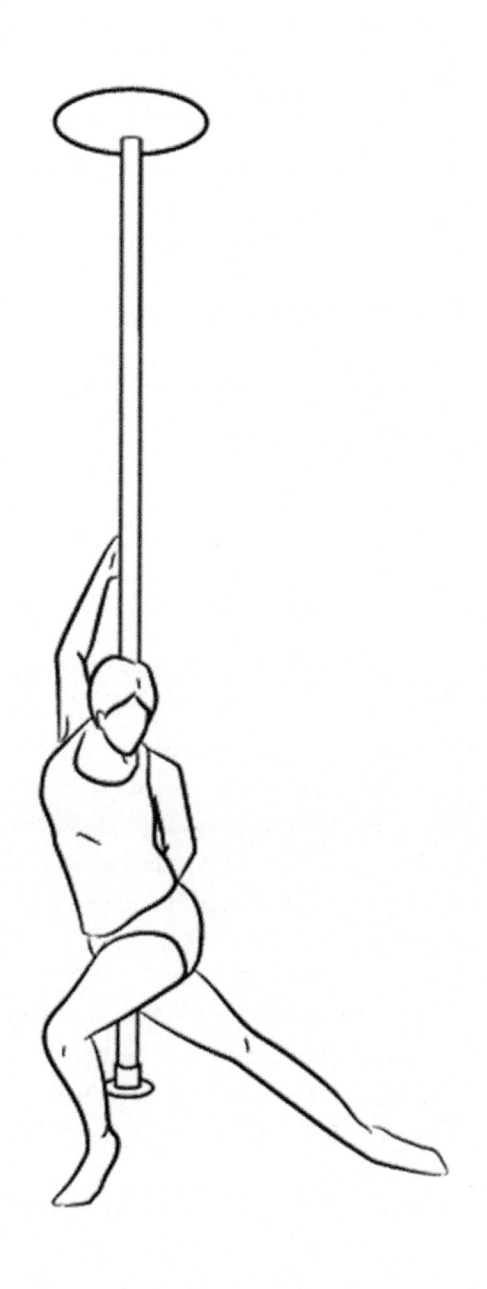

Transitional Moves and How to Do Them

Transitional moves are a great way to really hone your pole dancing skills. These are perfect for those who don't really have the strength just yet. Often, for beginners, you're using muscles you typically don't use, and these transitional moves are nice for not only segueing from one move to another but are also great to help you feel sexy as well. This chapter will go over transitional moves, what they are, and describe a few to help you get started.

What Are Transitional Moves?

Essentially, transitional moves are moves that allow you to transition from one move to another. For example, let's say that you are going from a spinning move to a climbing move. When you finish the spin, you might end up realizing it looks awkward going from one move to another. If you're considering doing this for performance, it's obvious to the audience when you're going to do one and then the other if you don't have a fitting transitional move. It also creates a sort of blank space in your routine, which could be filled by one of these moves.

These transitional moves are so simple anyone from a beginner to a veteran can do these. There are so many transitional moves, that they will be covered at further skill levels as well, but for learning beginner moves, this chapter will go over just a few of them to help you create great combinations.

Not only that, transitional moves are great to learn once you feel your arms burn out a little bit after doing lots of climbs and spins. Sure, you could do those moves all day and night but adding a few transitional moves here and there makes for smoother, sleeker combos.

Body Wave

This is the easiest and best transitional move for any beginner who's trying to perfect a way to transition from spinning to climbing. It's very simple and you don't have to do all that much. Plus, if you throw your head back and pop your booty, you'll end up looking really sexy.

To do the body wave finish your spin, and from there, start to straighten up. You should push your chest in the direction to the pole, and then thrust your hips, then your shoulders back, and then pull your hips forward once more. Repeat it again and again. You'll notice that it might look a bit weird at first, but when you do this in a more fluid manner, rather than just a bunch of separate moves, it creates a sort of wave motion, and it can look sexy.

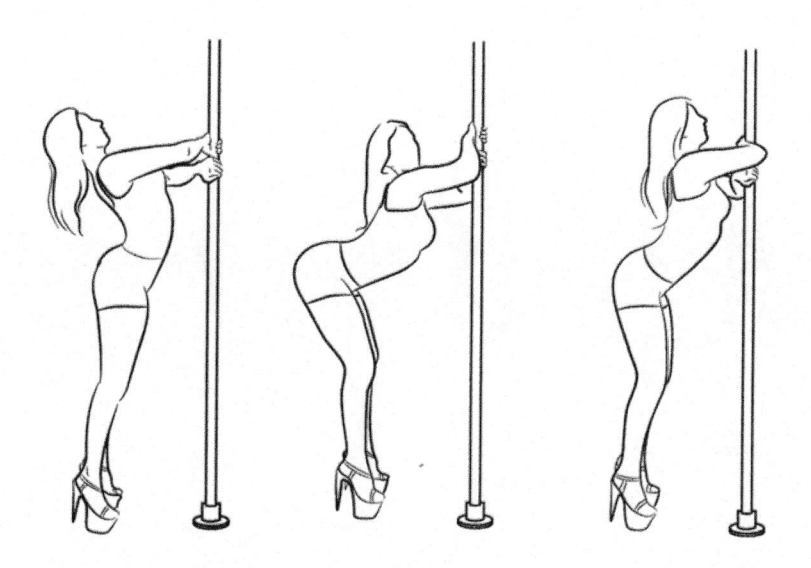

Backwards Wiggle

This is good to try after doing a basic walk-around and you want to add a bit of sexiness to your combo. To do this, get in front of the pole and stand up straight with your back next and touching it. You should then take the pole and hold it with both hands. Then, move your hips from one side to the other as you begin to lower your body into almost a crouching position. You should stop when your thighs are at about a 90-degree angle. From there, you can move your hands down, push your knees apart for just a moment, and then push them back up into a standing position.

For future combos — especially more advanced ones — this is a perfect transitional move to other mounts and it's a great beginner transition to learn to make any combo that much sexier.

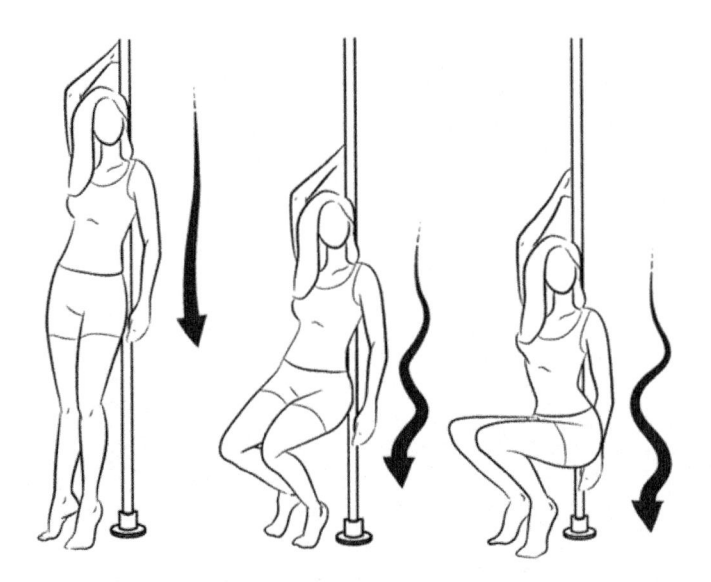

Pole Wiggles

While the name may seem silly to read, this is another great transitional move for those who are looking to try something to move from a spin to a climb. To do this, you should be facing the pole with your feet on each side, a little less than shoulder width apart. You should hold the pole just below your head with your dominant hand. Move your hips from one side to the other until you've crouched down. Once you're in the crouched position, you can push your dominant leg up and point the toes, and then move your hips back and start to push it up until you're standing once again.

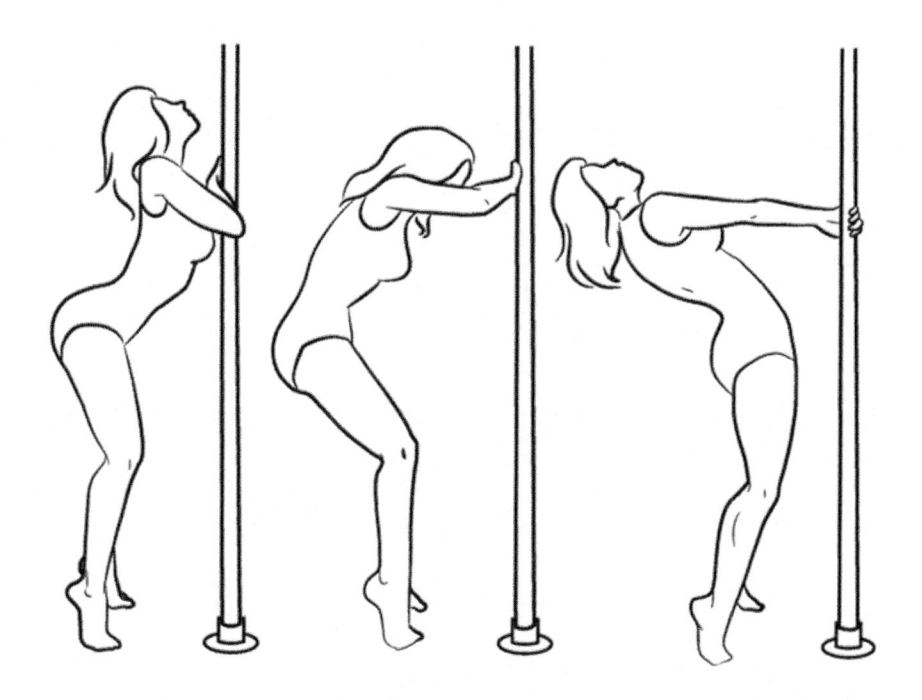

Hip Circles

This is a variation of the backward wiggle, in that you are once again standing with your back to the pole and your hands either above your head or on your hips. From there, you simply move your hips in a circle as you move down the pole. This is a very simple, but effective transitional move, especially for any shoulder movements later on.

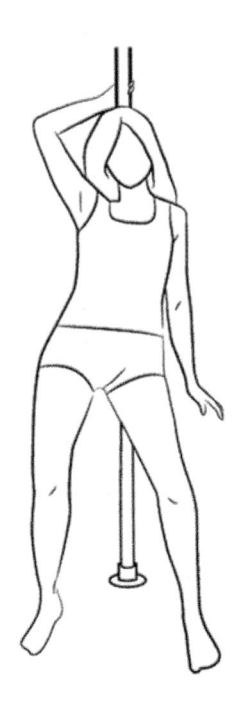

Pole Frisking

This is another variation of the basic wiggle, in that at first, you're facing the pole straight with your hands around it for support. To do this, you can bend your knees slightly back and forth, moving them in a sort of pointed manner. You should also bend at the waist, moving your body and your hands down the pole. This is a simple and yet very effective sort of transition — not only that — it adds a touch of extra sexiness!

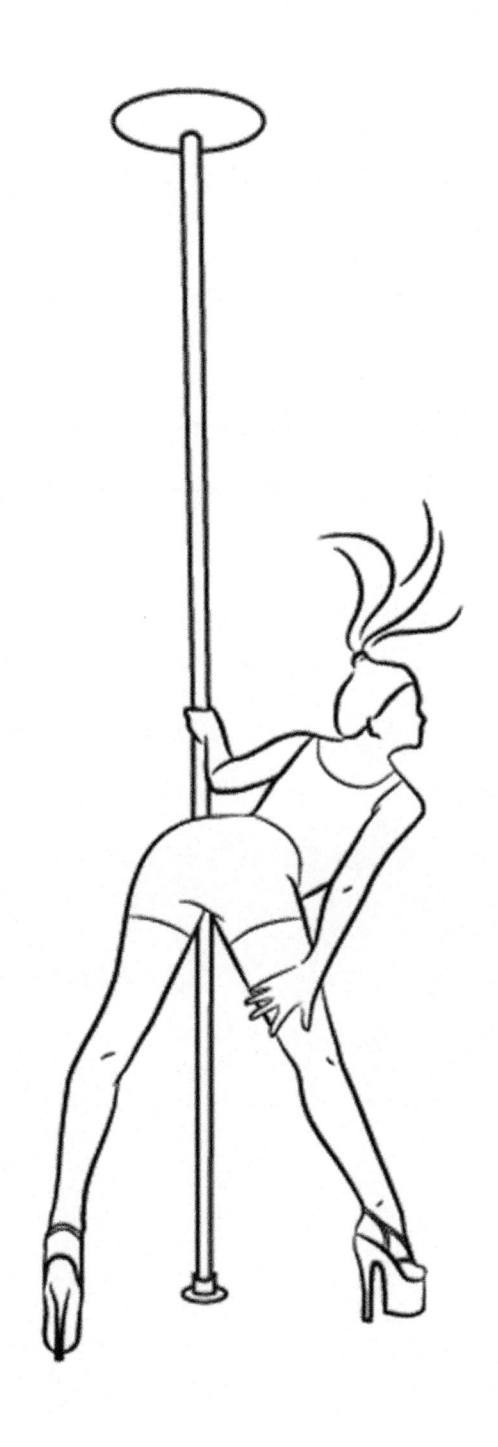

Knee Bridge

This is a good move if you're on the floor and you want to get back up on your feet without looking awkward. To do this, you need to be on the ground. Your legs should be next to one another with your knees spread a bit apart. From there, you should lean back as far as possible and grip the pole, if you so desire. You can then wrap your hands around the pole, propel yourself up, and move on to the next move. This is a great way as well to build up arm and abdominal strength and it'll improve flexibility as well.

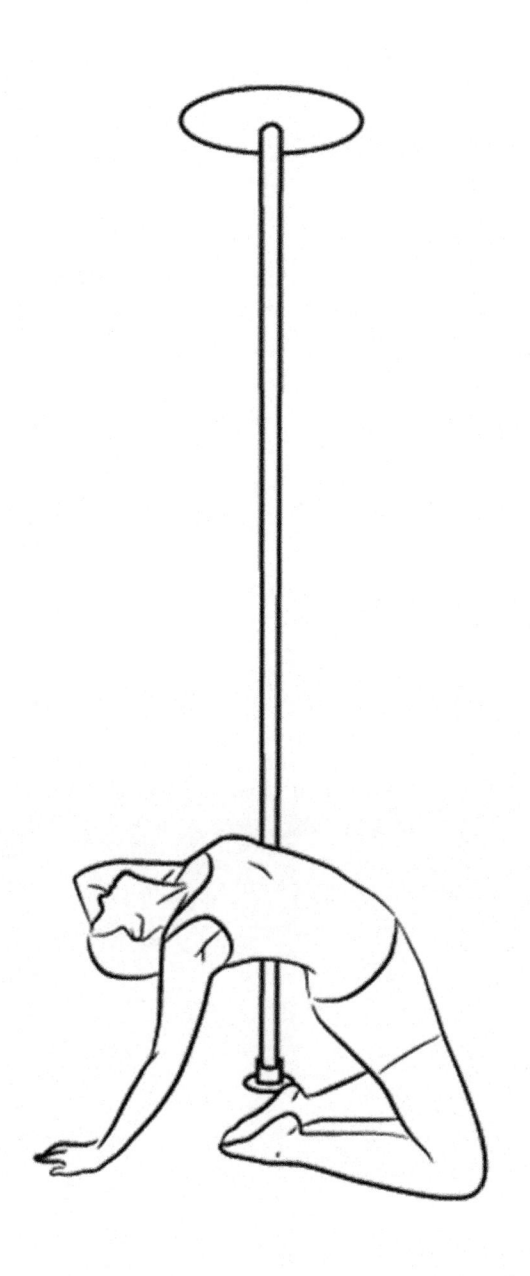

Shoulder Bridge

This is another great flexibility transition. To do this, you need to be on the ground. Move your feet up so that your toes are pointed, and your knees are bent, kind of like a bridge position. You then put your hands straight, moving them to each side, and holding the position there with your shoulders. You can grip the pole and pull yourself up from there. This is another great move to help build your strength and make you look sexy.

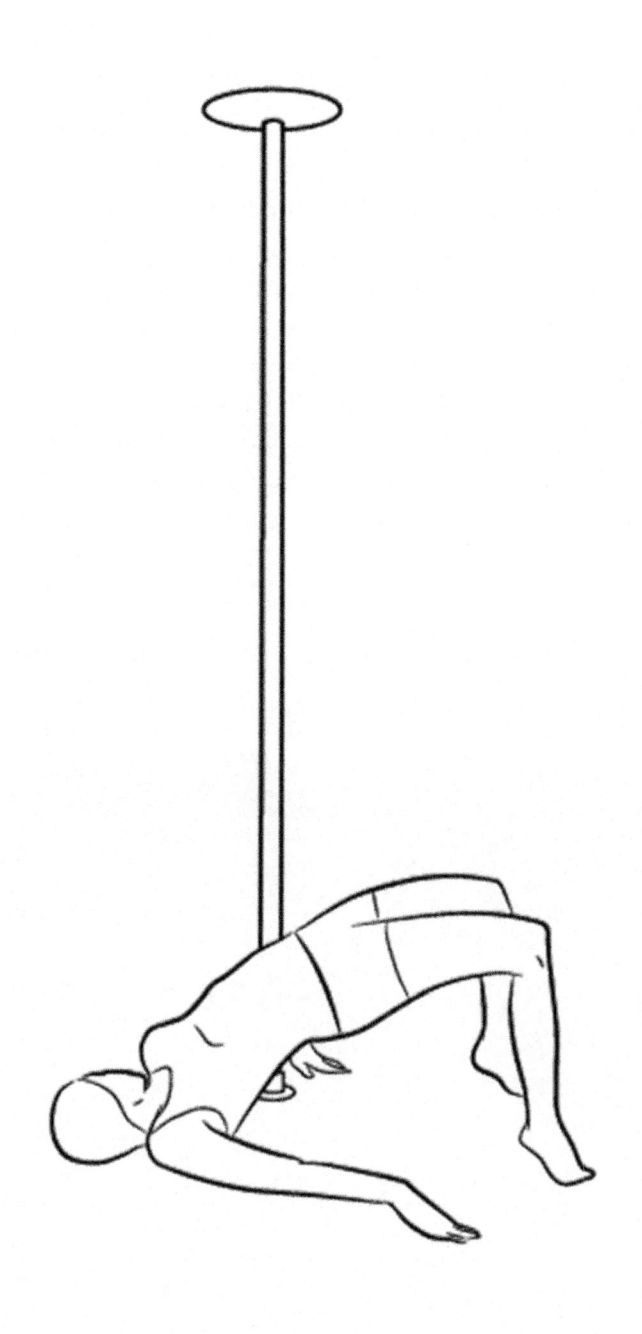

Clock Legs

This is another sexy and fun transitional move and it'll also look pretty once you've mastered it. In order to do this, you need to lie back on your elbows with your back and butt against the ground. Point your legs straight up to the sky and keep your toes pointed. Keep your knees together. You can then bend each leg one at a time and rotate it in a clockwise fashion. The real trick with this move, however, is keeping your legs pointed.

A common problem with many who begin pole dancing is that they don't keep their toes pointed. Pointed toes allow for a more beautiful and fluid motion of your legs and it doesn't look as jarring and awkward. Whenever you're doing a move, strive to keep those toes pointed unless otherwise specified.

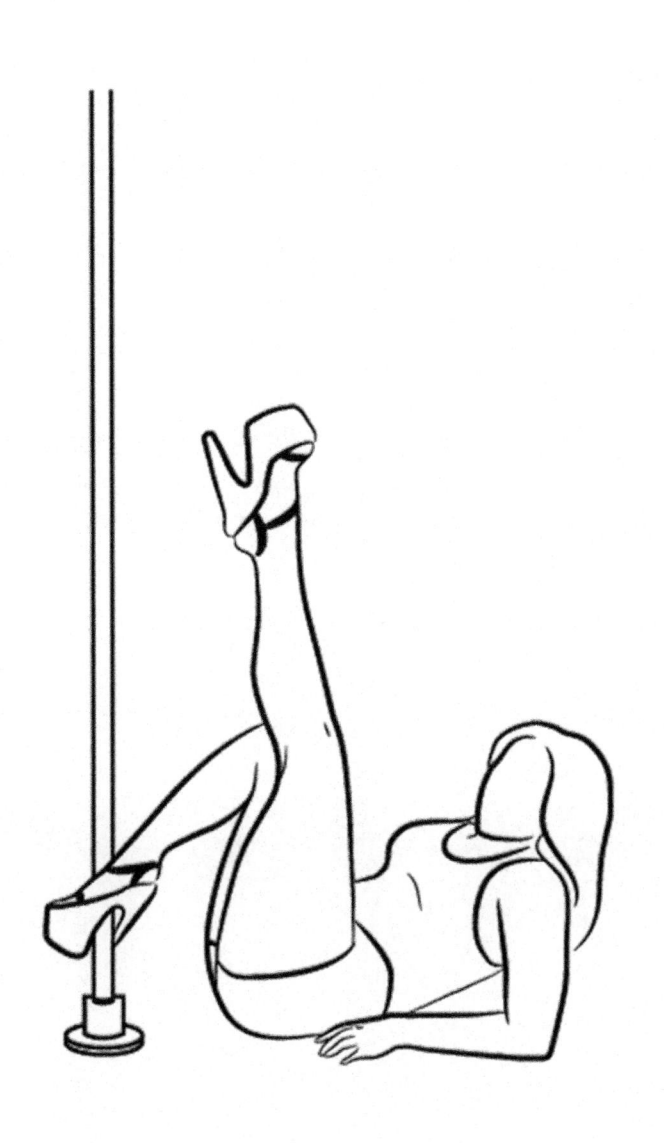

Log Roll

The final transitional move we'll go over is the log roll. To do this, you should lie on your back with your body near the pole. Grasp the pole and hold onto it, keeping a very strong grip. You should then take your upper body and move yourself to the other side, maintain pointed toes and also keep your back flat. This is very similar to a plank. This is also a great way to improve abdominal strength, which is integral to pole dancing.

These transitional moves are great for those beginning their pole dancing journey. Not only that but using them with various spins and other combos will allow you to have an even better routine and it will make you feel not only more confident but sexier.

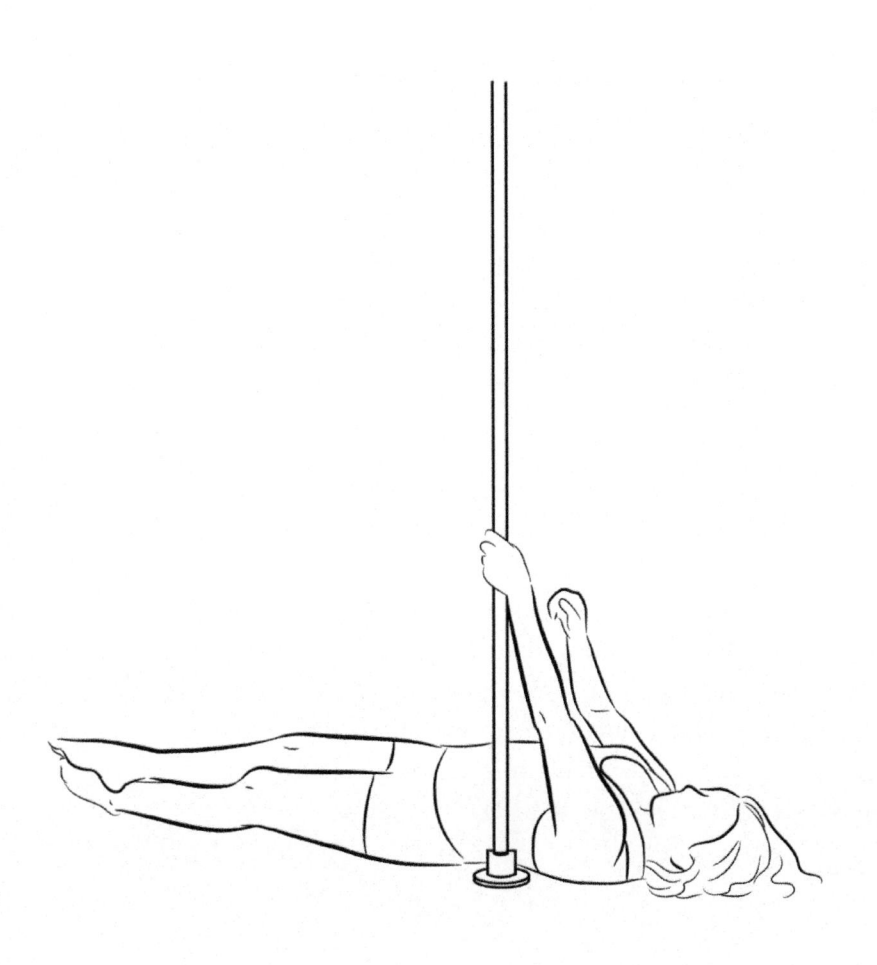

More Beginner Moves to Perfect and Learn

There are many beginner moves out there but these are the best ones to start with. Learning these will make your pole dancing abilities shine and while it does take a bit of time to get used to, you'll certainly enjoy each of them once you master them.

Hook Spin

With this move, you start by moving forward around the pole area with the arm inside holding the pole. From there, you take your inside leg and hook it against the front area of the pole and take your outside arm against the pole. You can then pull the outside leg up and into this position. It's a bit awkward at first and might take a minute to get used to, but once you do, this beginner spin is tons of fun.

43

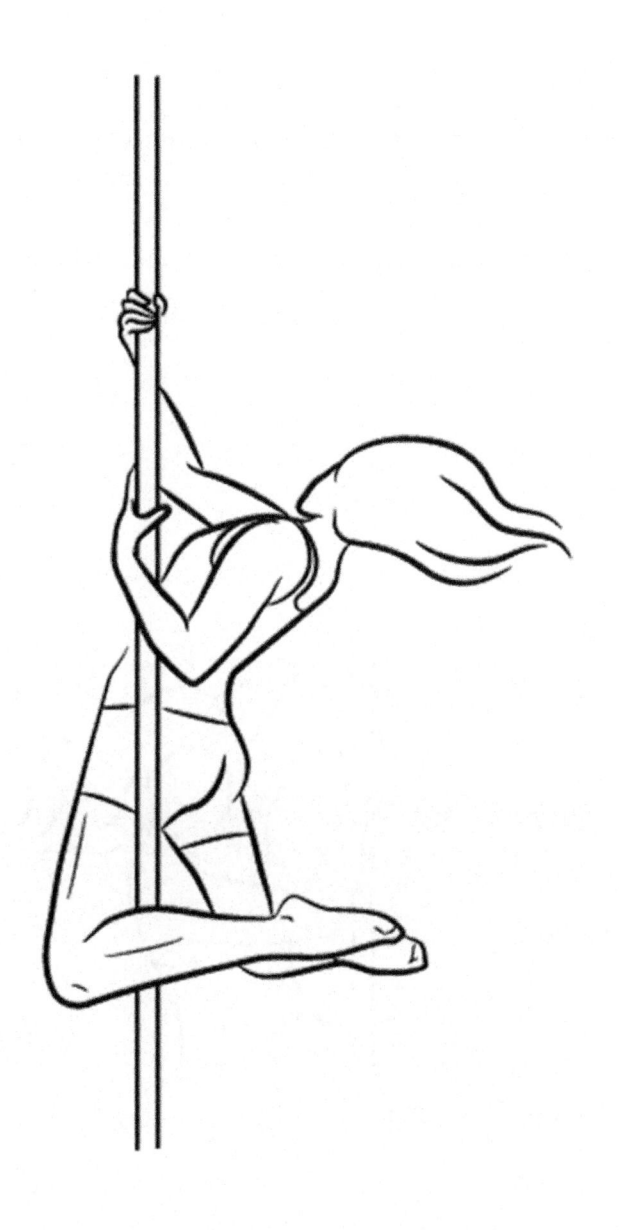

Martini

This is another great spin that's perfect for any beginner. To start, you should walk forward around the pole, making sure that your inside arm is holding the pole. You should then take the inner leg and put it in front and take your outside arm and put it on the pole. You will bring your outside leg to the pole last. You should then extend your leg and have it angled in an upward fashion. Make sure that when you do this you that point your toes for best results.

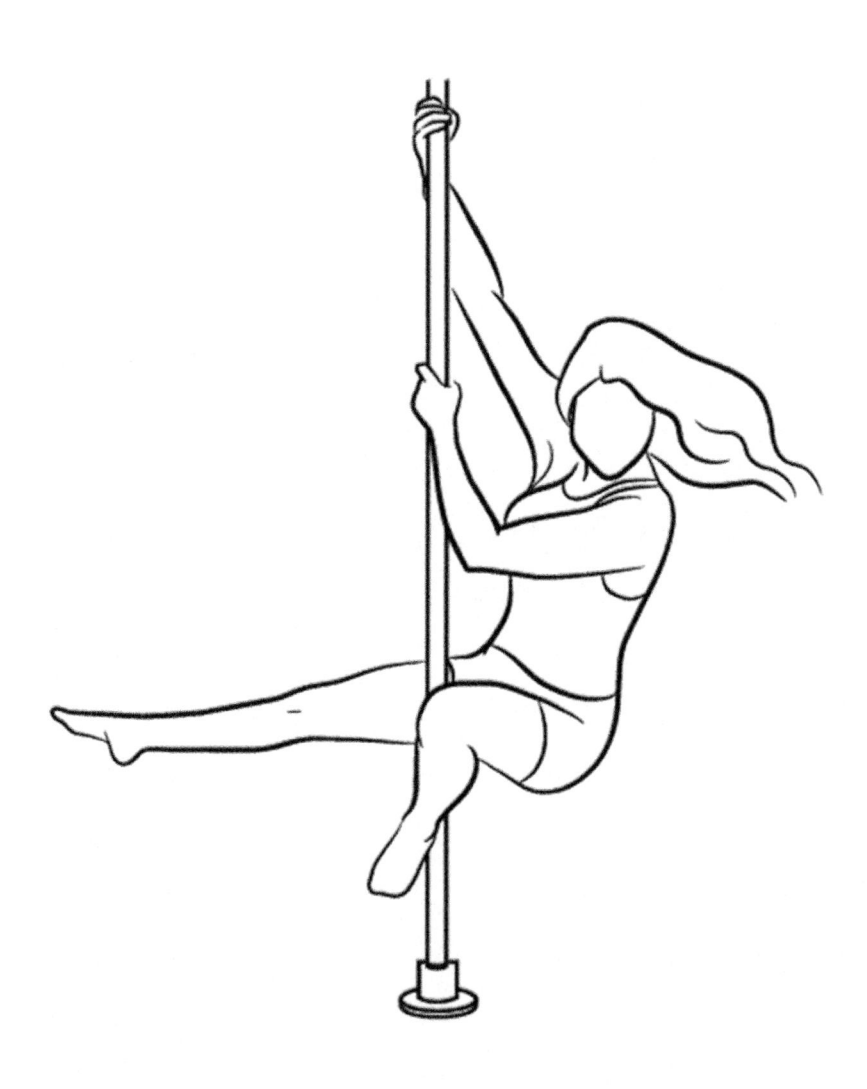

Chair Spin

This is a beginner move that looks deceptively easy, but it's actually designed to really build your strength. You need to have sufficient strength in your arms to do this, since you'll be supporting your body weight in one of your arms and you'll be holding yourself away with the other hand.

To do this, you take the dominant hand and put it above your head and on the inside of the pole, holding it there. Then, you take your outside hand and place it on the pole. You'll then push yourself up, holding both of your legs together, and strive to hold yourself there without touching the pole. Initially, you probably will need to touch the pole to maintain the grip, but once you get stronger, you'll be able to hold yourself further away from the pole, allowing you to create a pretty spin.

To really make this look clean, you should try to make sure that you have your knees bent together and try to make your body go slightly horizontal once you've mastered the initial moves. It takes a bit of skill, but once you've maintained it, you'll have no problems.

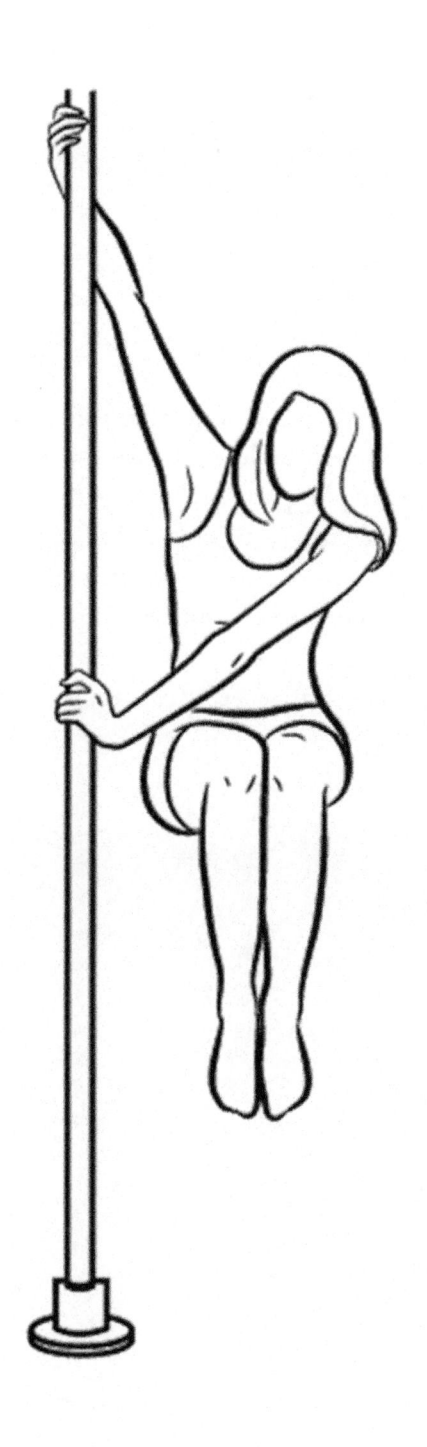

Pike Spin

This is essentially a variation of the chair spin. Instead of bending, you're essentially extending your legs out and holding them in that on. To do this, you should make sure that you have your dominant hand on the pole as before, with your shoulders down and working. You should use the outside leg to push yourself up, holding your body there as you swing out from the pole in a wide arc. Once you spin, you should use your inside hand to maintain your body away from where the pole is. You shouldn't grip the pole with this hand since it'll bring your body close to the pole and the spin won't work right. After lift-off, you should immediately keep the legs up, together, extended, and with the toes pointed. You can keep this spin going and once you decide to finish, you can then transition to a chair spin with your feet planted. You can keep doing this, again and again, working to hold your body away from the pole. This is a great move to build your core, hip flexors and even leg strength if you so desire. It's a fun, basic move that's relatively easy to learn.

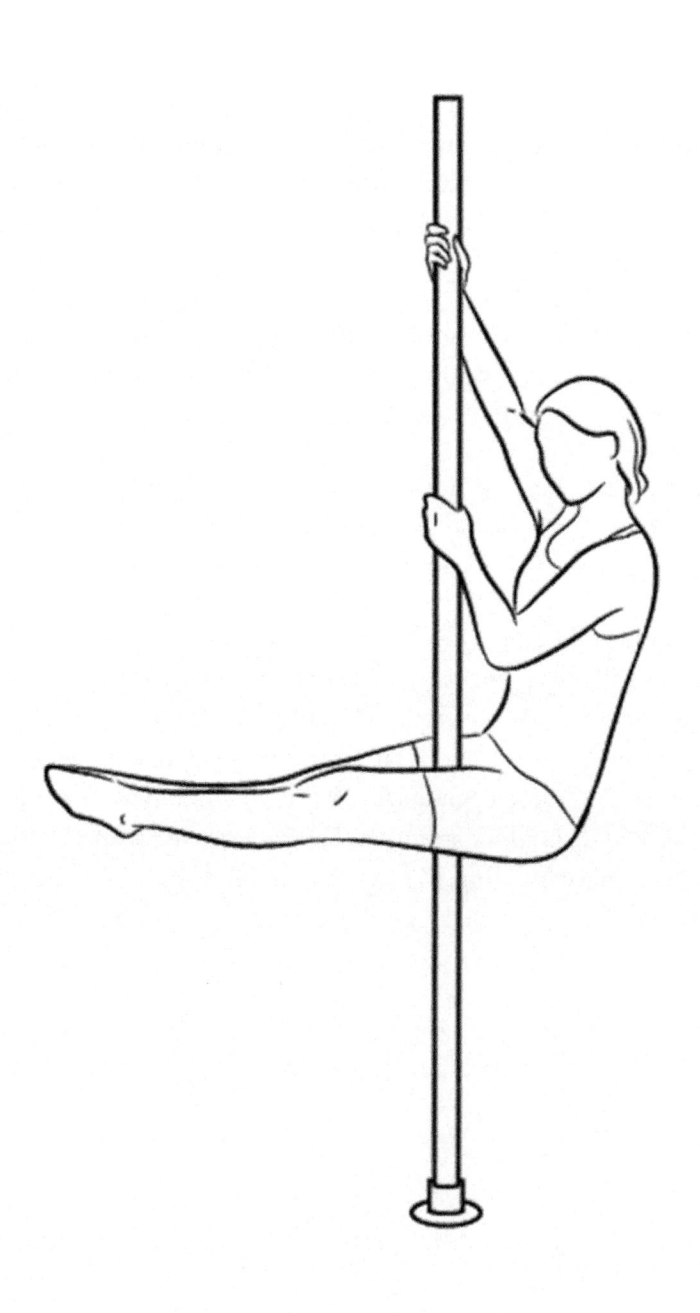

Back Hook Spin

This is also called a goddess spin. To start, you should start walking around the pole, wrapping your leg around, and from there, you will pivot your body around. From there, let your body almost fall. You can then grip the pole with your legs, slowly letting your body fall slightly.

This is much harder than the front hook spin, because many beginners often fear falling down on the pole. It's important that you learn the basic front hook spin before trying this move since it's a bit harder to let your body simply fall.

The biggest thing to remember is to not grip the pole super tight when you do move your body down. You should hold it just enough to create a fluid movement. Imagine holding a glass and then letting yourself go.

Contrary to what was said before, you should actually wear yoga pants with this move. The pants will help prevent you from sticking too much to the pole. Obviously, during a routine, you can't switch pants, but for practice, and to help make you feel more confident about falling, try wearing them to help ease your body into it. If you're still struggling with move, you should work to build your arms, core, back and shoulder strength. The rotator cuff is an area that will require a lot of strength building, so keep that in mind.

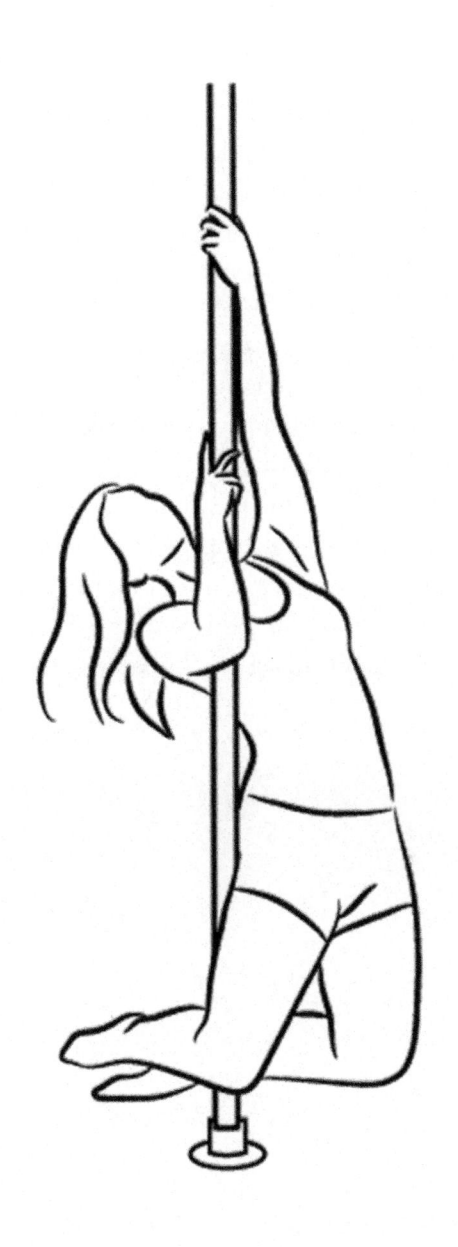

Stag Spin

This is another spin that is fun to do. It's also known as the ballerina or the sun wheel spin. Before you do this, you should learn both the fireman and the chair spins before moving on, especially since this one does require you to have precision and strength in your obliques. If you're not able to get your legs up to that position, it's best that you start to build up your abdominals first.

To do this move, you should first learn the leg placement. Your outside leg should hold the pole right where your Achilles tendon is. Your back leg will be bent and extended, almost lifted slightly. You should have the inner and more dominant hand up, while the outside hand is lower. To do this, you walk, and then wrap your outside leg around the pole, holding it with the Achilles tendon once more, and then lifting the other leg. You should then hold the position there. This might be a bit awkward, simply because you might not be used to this. You should then let your body simply fall to the ground naturally, allowing you to slide down and then move into a transitional move.

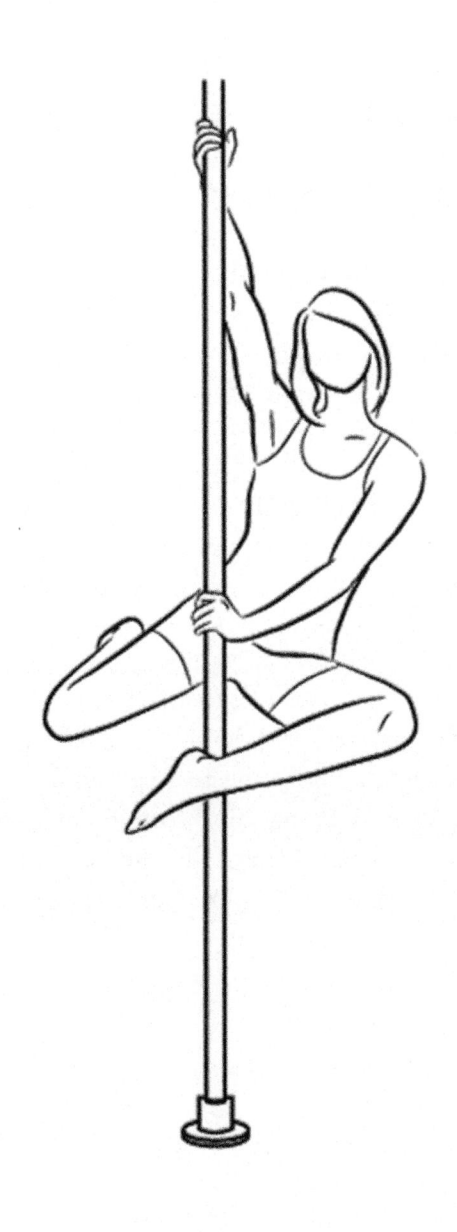

Crucifix Climb

This is similar to the basic climb, but instead of having your legs straight, one of them is bent, while the other one is straight. To do this, you begin with the dominant hand and leg against the pole, and then you lift off with this. You then bring up the weaker side — like your typical climb. From there, you slide one leg up and then the other and continue to do this. You should move the dominant hand up first, and then the weaker hand. You can continue to do this until you get to the top of the pole. Hold it there for a minute to build strength and to slide down, you simply release your legs slightly, holding the pole as you climb down.

Now that you know a bit more about the basic pole moves, it's time to work on them, perfect them and strive to add transitions and slides. All of these pole dancing moves can have any of the other transitions added to them, allowing you to create some neat combinations.

The best way to learn any of these moves is to take one, start to work on it and keep doing it until you begin to feel confident doing it. Often, if a move is very abdominally-focused, you might not be able to do it right away. The best thing to do is to add some supplement some core work to your workouts, to help your body perform these moves successfully. Remember, practice makes perfect, and with pole dancing, it certainly isn't an exception.

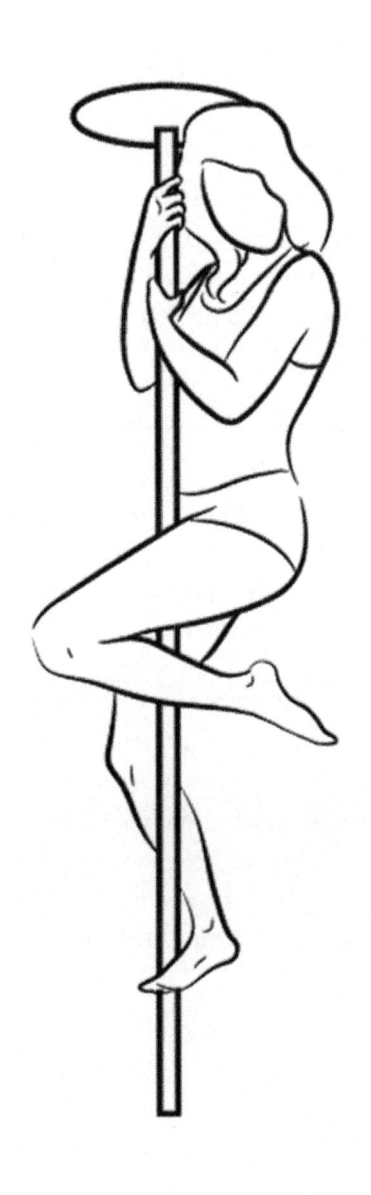

Go Shine!

As you've seen here, pole dancing is art. It's a fitness exercise, but also a creative means to really shine. While some people still associate pole dancing with strippers, it's not merely an activity for them anymore. Anyone can use it! Pole fitness is a ton of fun and you'll certainly love all of the confidence you'll start to ooze the minute you begin to try it!

Now, your next step is simple. Read over the material again each time you start to work on a new move. It's great to read it the first time, but make sure you have this book out before you start pole dancing. Make sure you prepare yourself for what you're about to do and from there, try it. Make sure to be safe. Don't have anything slick and slippery on and avoid baggy clothing. Try all of these moves and begin to learn them.

As an aside, you will probably not learn these moves right away. Most of these beginner moves take lots of practice. I remember when I began, it took me about 30 minutes just to get the fireman spin down. It's a bit of a struggle and initially, you might not even be able to hold yourself up for more than a couple of seconds. But don't despair. Instead, keep working at this, keep trying to push forward, and from there, you'll see the results! You'll see just how far you've come as you continue to practice this amazing form of art.

Win a free

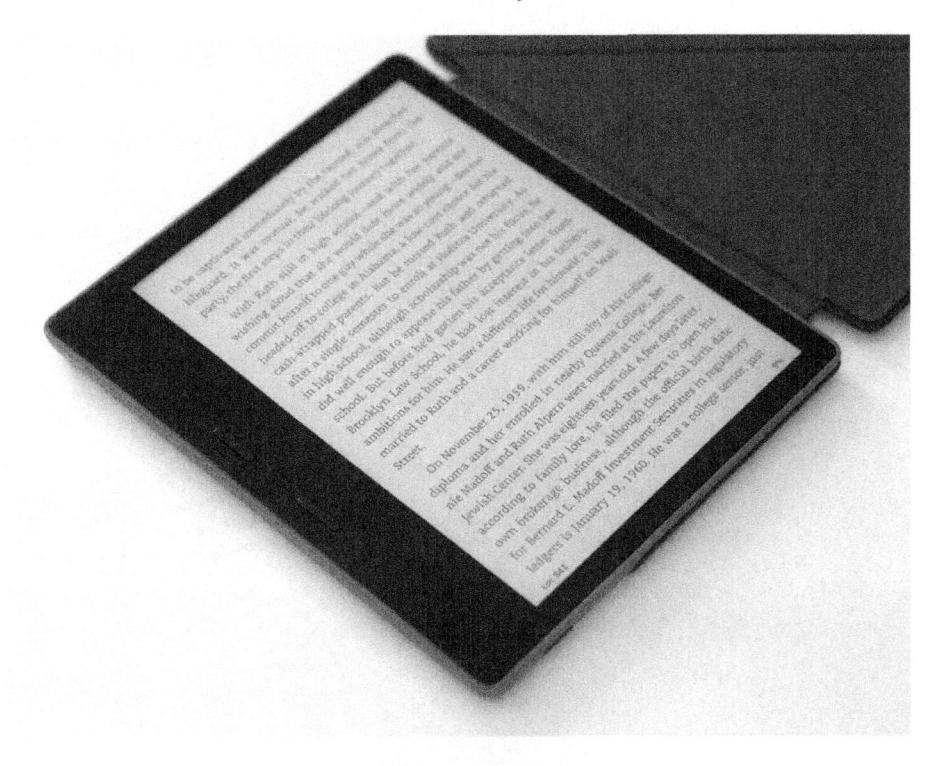

kindle
OASIS

Let us know what you thought of this book to enter the sweepstake at:

http://booksfor.review/beginnerpole

Want to take your pole dancing to the **next level**?

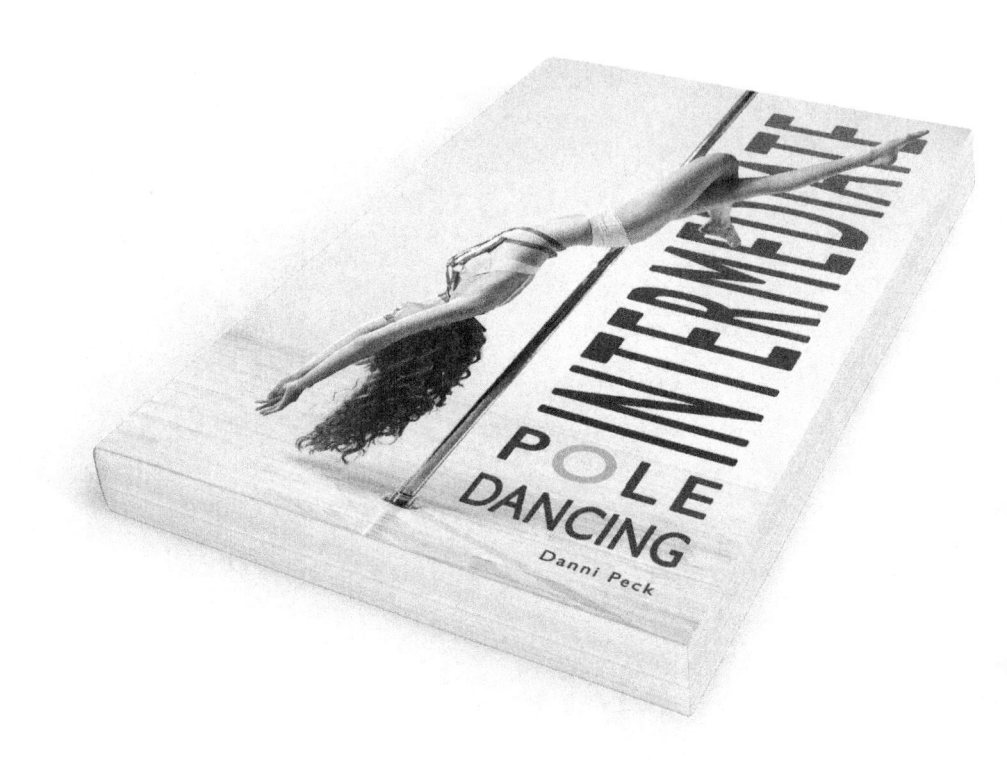

Intermediate Pole Dancing
For Fitness and Fun

Available on Amazon

Page intentionally left blank

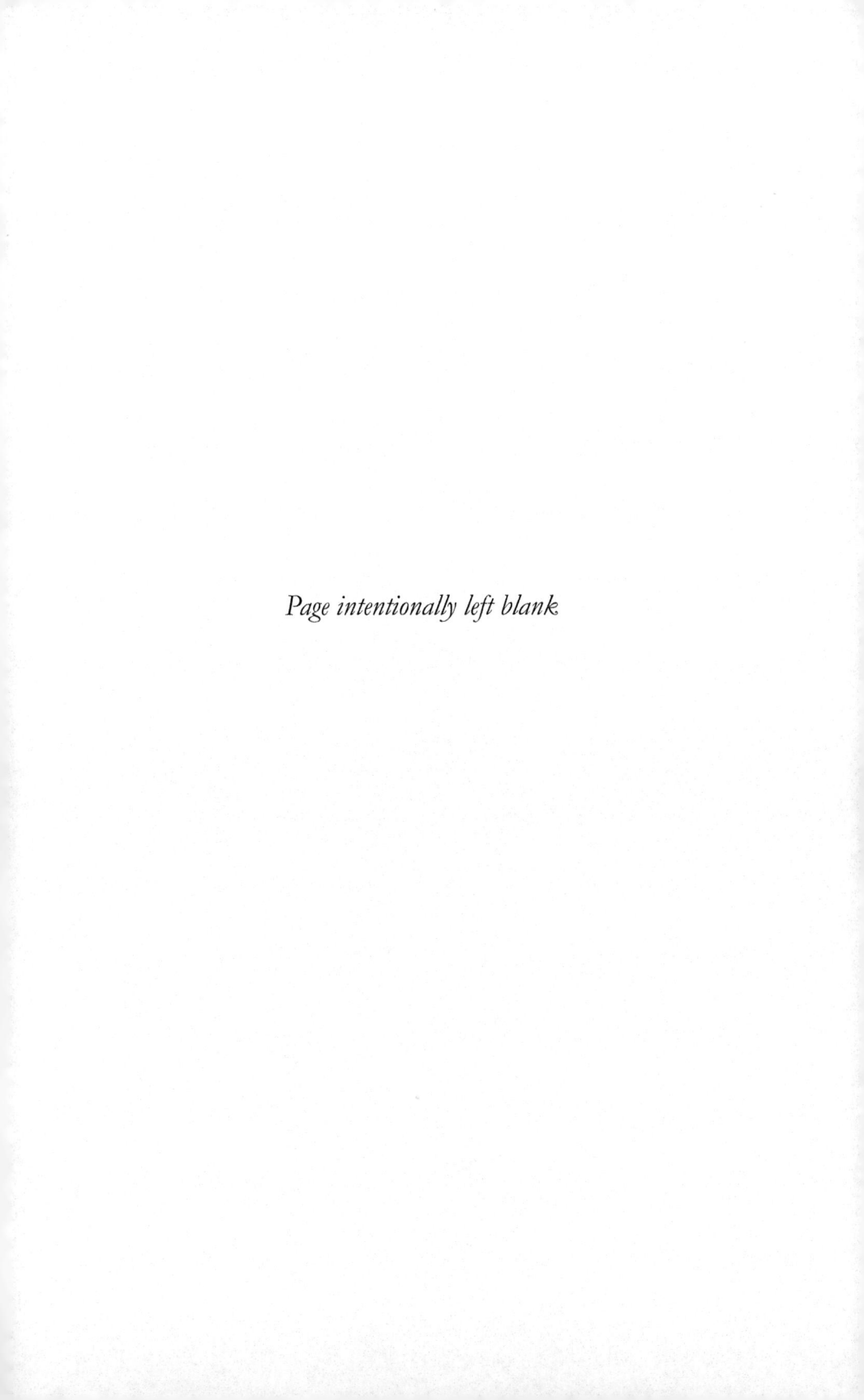

Printed in Great Britain
by Amazon